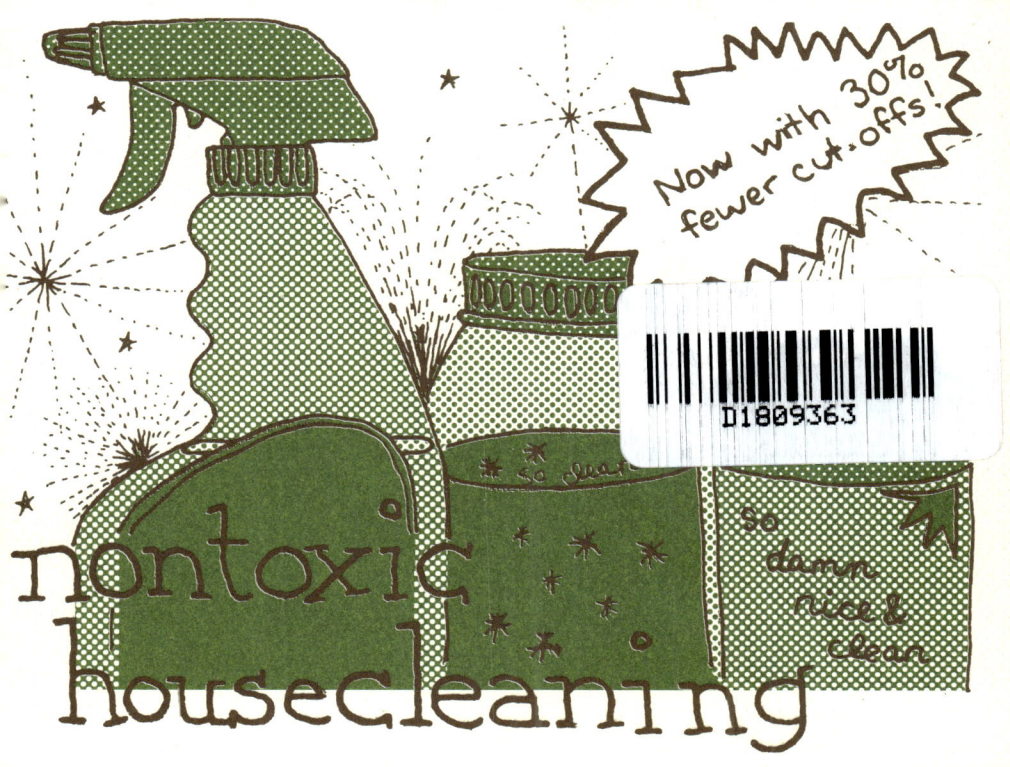

Now with 30% fewer cut-offs!

D1809363

so clean

so damn nice & clean

nontoxic

housecleaning

This is a zine I made to accompany a Nontoxic Housekeeping workshop I led during a summer DIY workshop series. Here's a selected bibliography:

- The Naturally Clean Home (Karyn Siegel Maier)
- Herbal Homekeeping (Sandy Maine)
- SOLVE IT WITH SALT! (Patty Moosbrugger)
- Natural Cleaning For Your Home (Casey Kellar)
- VIM AND VINEGAR! (Melodie Moore)
- BAKING SODA BONANZA! (Peter E. Ciullo)

So what's the point of DIY cleaning when you can buy dozens of beautifully packaged, expensive and totally toxic products at your local supermarket? The answer's in the question I suppose, but here are a few more very good reasons to DIY:

· Making your own cleaners saves you money, especially since every ingredient I include can be used for many, many other things besides cleaning.

· Every time you make and use a homemade product, Procter + Gamble make less money!

· You don't have to worry about kids, animals, or stupid friends getting poisoned by Drano or Lysol or whatever.

· You can scrub your whole house, without gloves and without corrosive burns & blisters. Score!

· Fewer chemicals means less contamination of grey-water, groundwater, and indoor air.

# Quick Tips

• Add ½ c vinegar or lemon juice to dishwater to cut grease. For stuck-on food, scrub with baking soda while the dish/pan is still hot. You can also boil a solution of 1 c water + 3 T baking soda in the dirty pan. Let sit until the food can be scraped off.

• Get grease spots off rugs using 1 part salt + 3 parts rubbing alcohol

• Clean the fridge with a solution of ½ c water, 3 T baking soda, and 6 drops essential oil of your choice

• Get rid of fridge demons by placing ½ c coffee grounds in a bowl on a fridge shelf. You can also string bundles of fresh herbs from the wire racks

• Sprinkle baking soda in garbage cans, litter boxes, and down drains to deodorize.

Here's a list of stuff that comes in handy when you are making your own science. I selfishly excluded the ingredients listed in other recipes I've found that I think are gross (gelatin, bleach, caustic acids):

- vinegar (cheap + white, unless specified)
- baking soda
- borax (sounds scary, but it's not)
- salt
- lemon juice
- washing soda
- ammonia (kind of gross, but meh)
- castile soap (a very gentle + kind tallow-free soap. Try Dr. Bronner's liquid or Kirk's for grating.)

- essential oils (different oils serve different purposes. I will elaborate on this later.)
- dried herbs like rosemary, thyme and oregano

- You'll also need measuring cups + spoons, funnels, a mixing utensil (plastic or stainless steel) and all sorts of containers. Keep this stuff separate from what you use to make food.

# Essential Oils

Always use pure essential oils when you're making cleaners at home. Don't use anything labeled "perfume oil" or "aromatherapy oil." Essential oils can retain some of the antimicrobial, antibacterial, and antiviral properties of the whole plant. Here are some oils that come in useful:

- <u>Antibacterial</u>: bay, camphor, cardamom, chamomile, citronella, cypress, eucalyptus, ginger, hyssop, juniper, lavender, lemon, lemongrass, lemon verbena, lime, marjoram, orange, pine, rosemary, sage, sandalwood, spearmint, tea tree, thyme

- <u>Antimicrobial</u>: bergamot, chamomile, clove, eucalyptus, hyssop, lavender, lemon, lime, myrtle, nutmeg, oregano, patchouli, tea tree

- <u>Antiviral</u>: cinnamon, eucalyptus, lavender, lemon, oregano, sandalwood, tea tree, thyme

**\* DON'T INGEST ESSENTIAL OILS!**

# General Cleaners

*for all your vague cleaning needs*

## Eucalyptus, Lavender, & Tea Tree Oil Spray Cleaner

1 t liquid castile soap

1 t borax

¼ t eucalyptus e.o.

3 drops tea tree e.o.

2 T white vinegar

2 c hot water

¼ t lavender e.o.

• Mix all ingredients together in a spray bottle. Use on any surface except glass. To use, spray on, scrub, and rinse off with a clean, damp towel or cloth.

## Eucalyptus-Mint All-Purpose Disinfecting Soft Soap

5 c grated castile soap

½ c baking soda

1 t borax

6 c hot peppermint tea

1 t eucalyptus essential oil

• Put grated soap into a 3 qt. stainless steel saucepan + add tea. Simmer 15 minutes on low heat. Add remaining ingredients. Store in a jug or squirt bottle. Shake before using.

## Carpet Cleaner

3 c water
3/4 c liquid castile
2-3 drops peppermint
essential oil
· Mix all ingredients
in a blender. Rub
foam into carpet
with a damp sponge.
Let dry + then vacuum.
\* If your carpet
just smells funny,
sprinkle the
carpet with equal
parts borax and
baking soda, and
then vacuum.

## Wood Floors

1½ c water
1½ c vinegar
20 drops peppermint
essential oil
· Combine all
ingredients in a
spray bottle. Use
sparingly, working
on small sections
of the floor.
Dry mop after
using.

## Vinyl + Tile Floors

### Actually Lemony
1 c liquid castile soap
1/4 c lemon juice
1/4 eyedropper tea
tree essential oil
6 c warm water
· Mix all ingredients +
store in a plastic jug.

### Actually Pine-y
1 c liquid castile soap
1/2 c pine oil or extract
6 c warm water
· Mix all ingredients
+ store in a plastic
jug.

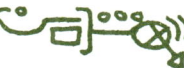

## Wall Cleaner

1 c vinegar
1 gallon water
• & that's it! Combine in a bucket and apply with a sponge

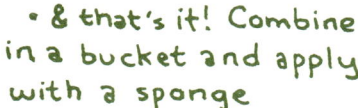

## Spray-On Fabric Cleaning

1 c water
⅛ c liquid soap
½ t baking soda
1 T vinegar
• Combine in a spray bottle. Spray on, scrub with a sponge and blot well with a damp cloth.

## Gentle Wood Cleaner

½ c canola oil
¼ c liquid castile soap
¼ c water
• Combine + shake well before using (mix will want to separate). Apply with a rag, finish with a dry rag + follow with polish.

## "Dry Clean" for Upholstery

½ c baking soda
½ c cornstarch
• Make into a paste with some water. Apply to fabric, let sit 30 minutes. Brush off with a stiff-bristled brush. Vacuum seriously.

## Gentle Window Cleaner

3 t liquid soap    3/4 c white vinegar    1/2 t baking soda

• Combine all ingredients in a spray bottle. Shake well before using. Use old newspapers instead of paper towels.

## Lemon-Mint Window Wash

Juice of 1 lemon   2 c water or club soda  1/2 t peppermint oil* 1 t cornstarch

• Follow instructions for Gentle Window Cleaner.

## Mirror Cleaner

1 1/2 c vinegar    1/2 c water   8 drops any citrus e.o.

• Combine all ingredients in a spray bottle. Shake well before using. Spray on + wipe off with a cloth or crumpled newspapers.   * use peppermint <u>essential oil</u>, not <u>extract</u>!

# Dishes, Sinks & Drains

## Liquid Dish Soap - not for automatic dishwashers!

• Combine 22 oz. liquid castile soap with up to 30 drops essential oil of your choice. Shake well to blend. Citrus oils are purty-smelling and are effective degreasers, too.

## Basic Sink Cleanser - foamy!

¼ c baking soda    ½ c vinegar    3 drops essential oil

• Apply to a wet sink, scrub, and rinse with hot water.

## Herbal Scrubber -

*if you're using this in a tub or sink, you might want to put cheesecloth over the drain to catch the herby bits. Then make pizza!*

½ c baking soda    ½ c dried sage    ¼ c dried rosemary

• Combine in a jar + use like any scouring powder

## Drain Opener

• Pour 1 c each salt + baking soda, plus ½ c vinegar down the drain. Let sit 15 minutes, then flush it down with 2 quarts boiling water.

## Tub & Tile Soft Scrub

1 c baking soda   ¼ c liquid castile   3-5 drops tea tree oil
2 vitamin C or aspirin tablets, crushed fine

• Add water to make a paste. Scrub with a sponge + rinse thoroughly.

## Toilet Cleaner

2 c water   ¼ c liquid soap   1 T tea tree oil
10 drops eucalyptus or peppermint oil

• Combine well in a spray bottle. Spray on toilet + wipe off.

## Bowl Cleaner

½ c baking soda   ¼ c vinegar   10 drops tea tree oil

• Combine all ingredients, preferably in a papier maché volcano. Pour into toilet bowl & scrub.

## All-Purpose Laundry Soap

½ c baking soda    ½ c powdered castile soap    ¼ c borax
¼ c washing soda

- Mix ingredients well; use about ½ c per load of laundry

## Fabric Softener Sachet

yes, i said sachet.

½ c baking soda    1 T arrowroot powder    1-3 drops e.o.
1 T rice flour or cornstarch

- Mix ingredients well and place a few spoonfuls inside a sachet of <u>tightly woven</u> fabric. Tie tightly + add to dryer cycle. Refill the sachet when the scent fades.

## Homemade Bleach - store in a jug

1 c hydrogen peroxide    3 T lemon juice    15 c water

## Spray Starch - keep in a spray bottle. Mix well + use on light fabric.

3 T + 1 t cornstarch    4 c warm water

# Miscellaneous Recipes

## All-Purpose Desk & Equipment Duster Spray - oily!

| | |
|---|---|
| 1 c sweet almond oil | 2 T liquid soap |
| 2 T isopropyl alcohol | 1½ c water |

• Keep in a spray bottle. Spray on + Wipe off!

## Lemon Metal Cleaner (for brass + copper)

• Dip half a lemon in salt & rub it over copper. Wash with soapy water, rinse + buff dry.

## Oven Cleaner

• Scrub a COLD oven with equal parts vinegar and water.

## Appliance Cleaner - Unplug your toaster first!!!!

½ c vinegar    ½ c lemon juice    ¼ c water

• Mix together and keep refrigerated. Let sit on stains and scrub with a sponge.

Thanks so much for reading.
I love you.

Raleigh Briggs
letsgiveuptheghost@gmail.com

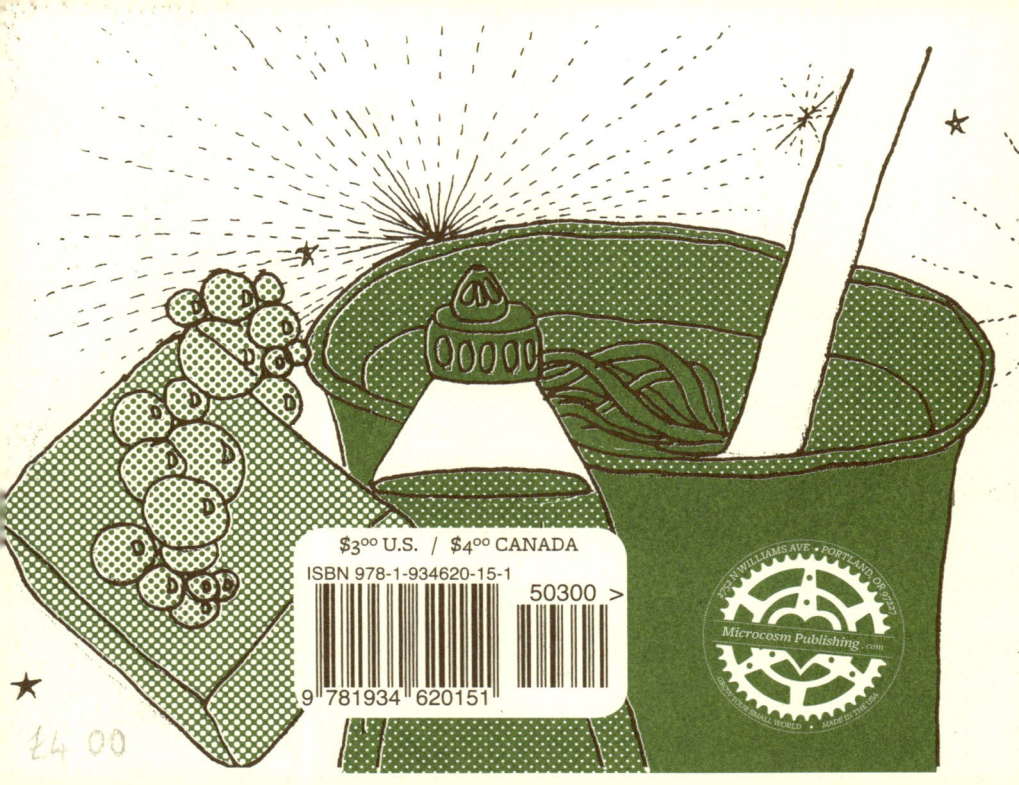

$3⁰⁰ U.S. / $4⁰⁰ CANADA

ISBN 978-1-934620-15-1

50300 >

9 781934 620151

£4 00